Praise

'This is not just a book; it is a manifesto for change, a call to arms for those of us committed to the service of humanity, and a handbook for the social work social entrepreneur. I urge you to delve into its pages, for within them lies the blueprint for a future where social work and entrepreneurship walk hand in hand, creating pathways to a better world.'

– **Vince Peart**, Independent Social Worker and Content Editor for *Social Work News*

'I found *Social Work and Beyond* an engaging and enjoyable read. It was inspiring to learn about the author's journey to becoming a social worker; he shares with the reader some of the most intimate and challenging times in his life. It is a book therefore, which is very much written in the first person. Equally, I appreciate Buturo's honesty in appraising the social work role today, both in terms of its rich rewards but also the huge demands it places on individuals, resulting sadly in many exiting the profession prematurely.

'Buturo describes reaching a crossroads in his social work career and needing to decide his next steps. It is evident that his transition to "social work entrepreneur", in terms of acquiring supported accommodation for young people and latterly a residential children's home, was a return to his roots as a residential worker. Buturo makes some persuasive arguments about social workers running successful businesses as opposed to private equity companies, who have very different motives for acquiring residential children's homes.

'Finally, there are thousands of social workers often referred to as independent social workers who are responsible for running their own businesses. This requires a different skillset which Buturo discusses in his book. This may not be a career choice to suit all social workers, but it is something that needs to be recognised as an option in career progression and, essentially, how social workers can become ethical entrepreneurs if this is the pathway they want to pursue. Social work and entrepreneurship need not be strange bedfellows if they accord with the values and principles of our profession.'

– **Nushra Mansuri**, Assistant Professor Academic, School of Psychological, Social and Behavioural Sciences, Coventry University

'I thoroughly enjoyed this book. It's an important useable contribution to our field and one I recommend as a must-read. It's full of valuable insights and practical knowledge underpinned by a hope and optimism only a great social worker could bring. I wish I'd had this resource when I ventured into the "business" side of social work.'

– **Dr Beverley Barnett-Jones MBE**, Associate Director (Practice and Impact), Nuffield Foundation

'*Social Work and Beyond* provides a really helpful and honest insight into the profession. Anyone who is thinking about branching out or changing direction would really benefit from Peter's words of wisdom.'

– **Sara Scholey**, Senior Consultant for Children's Transformation at Cumberland Council

Social Work and Beyond

How to be
a conscious
social work
entrepreneur

PETER NDUWAYESU BUTURO

Re think

First published in Great Britain in 2024 by Rethink Press (www.rethinkpress.com)

© Copyright Peter Nduwayesu Buturo

All rights reserved. No part of this publication may be reproduced, stored in or introduced into a retrieval system, or transmitted, in any form, or by any means (electronic, mechanical, photocopying, recording or otherwise) without the prior written permission of the publisher.

The right of Peter Nduwayesu Buturo to be identified as the author of this work has been asserted by him in accordance with the Copyright, Designs and Patents Act 1988.

This book is sold subject to the condition that it shall not, by way of trade or otherwise, be lent, resold, hired out, or otherwise circulated without the publisher's prior consent in any form of binding or cover other than that in which it is published and without a similar condition including this condition being imposed on the subsequent purchaser.

First and foremost, I have to thank God for the opportunity and wisdom to complete this book.

This book is dedicated to my mother, Mary Buturo, who tragically passed away in a car crash when I was sixteen years old. I miss my mother endlessly and I am forever thankful for her love towards me.

Contents

Foreword	1
Introduction	5
PART ONE Challenges	**11**
1 Meeting The Demands	**13**
The nature of social work	15
Multi-agency collaboration	19
Challenges	23
Accountability	27
Roles and responsibilities	29
My story	31
Summary	35
2 Honing Your Skills	**37**
Organisation and planning	39
Communication	47
Resilience	52
Summary	58

3 Preparing Yourself	**61**
Self-evaluation	62
Training	65
Learning	66
Discipline	67
Avoiding burnout	68
Achieving a work/life balance	71
Finding your why	74
Case studies	76
Top tips	78
Summary	80
PART TWO Opportunities	**83**
4 Taking The Leap	**85**
Have I reached my ceiling?	86
Do I have a vision?	87
Are my skills transferable?	88
Investing in yourself	90
What are my options?	92
What will it take?	101
Summary	103
5 Making It Happen	**105**
Knowing the market	106
Achieving visibility	106

Assembling a team		109
Working out the finances		110
Finding premises		115
Negotiating the legalities		118
Summary		120
6	**Living Your Purpose**	**123**
	Enjoy the challenge(s)	124
	Let go of the reins	127
	Take your time	128
	Trust the process	129
	Create a legacy	129
	Summary	130
Conclusion		**133**
Notes		**135**
Acknowledgements		**139**
The Author		**141**

Foreword

Are you a social worker? Have you left the profession, are you feeling at a crossroads, or perhaps even considering leaving? Or are you still on the increasingly stretched frontline, carrying scars from your practice experience, feeling that the resources and time you need to do the job well are increasingly limited? Regardless of your area of practice and how long you've been practising, if you are seeking practical and achievable ways of going beyond surviving in your role and learning to thrive within it – this is the book for you.

Part self-help, part sharing of his experience, and part basic business guide, this unique book is written by a social worker who clearly broadcasts his intentions. In over thirty-two years of experience working with children and families in need, I have never encountered a book for social workers as real-world, practical and accessible for both newcomers to the profession and those of us still here.

Though I enjoyed my consultancy work, at the time I lacked a business orientation. Peter helps you see that venturing into business as a social worker in the social care sector can build on your values and expand your influence. It can be a path, if you choose to leave frontline practice, which doesn't negate all the investment made in you, and by you, as a practitioner. Rather, it provides a livelihood to support yourself and family while employing others similarly in a role where your values and skills can still be fully utilised. Although it's not an easy transition to make, Peter shares concrete advice and insights to avoid the pitfalls ahead.

This book is truthful and honest about the waters we are collectively swimming in, and where the state stands in providing critical care for children who need it. These waters are not without controversy, which Peter openly tackles, making his argument that if there is to be 'profit' in care provision, as there already is, does society prefer committed, caring, accountable social work entrepreneurs leading in this space, or some offshore invisible equity where the risks of withdrawal are high? Peter knows where he stands.

Peter's love and care for social work and social workers abounds. I know this because throughout each chapter he tells us that social work is a higher calling. As Peter references, it's a worldwide profession uniquely placed in human services that supports, assists and confronts not only the personal challenges individuals face in their social living, but also the social structural challenges such as poverty and discrimination that impact that social living. He knows that doing this work requires an adaptive, empathetic and dynamic human and, to do it well, that person must care for themselves, and be cared for, to care well for others.

Purposefully written for social workers of today, in accessible prose, Peter's book lays out wisdom gained from his experience and absorbed from others. Tips for staying well, from organising the diary to a healthy sleep routine are never too few or far between. He writes about the necessary qualities for thriving in social work, such as (self-) discipline and finding positive support networks and a continued commitment to learning.

This book is a genuine call to stay in the profession, whether continuing on the 'job' or expanding the horizons of what you can do as a social worker, including the inspirational journey Peter is on from social work practitioner to CEO.

> **– Dr Beverley Barnett-Jones MBE,**
> Associate Director (Practice and Impact), Nuffield Foundation

Introduction

Social work is challenging. Having to deal with crises every day can make you feel as if you are inside a pressure cooker. It is a dark and lonely place, and at times you feel that it is a matter of fight or flight. I know. I have been there.

But the role of a social worker is powerful and important and much needed in our society. It is a position of trust that should not be undervalued.

My purpose in writing *Social Work and Beyond* is to remind you of the reasons you wanted to be a social worker and to outline the principles that will help you to survive and thrive in a profession that needs you. I want to encourage you by showing that there is light at the end of the tunnel, by providing you with a pathway towards self-awareness and balance – because the truth is that, to be able to take care of the children and families you work with, you must first take care of yourself. And I want to inspire you to make positive changes in your life and your career.

You might be thinking about becoming a social worker because you want to be an agent for change, to contribute to social justice and reform, to advocate for those who have no voice and stand up for those who don't have the ability to stand up for themselves. Or you might have years of practice behind you, but feel that you have hit a ceiling or reached your limit and gone as far as you possibly can. I have had that feeling many times as the workload became excessive and it felt that the world was on my shoulders.

Once you have read *Social Work and Beyond*, you will have the power of choice: the choice to continue as you are, or to make positive changes in the way you think, feel and act that will lead you to an explosion of opportunities that would not have been available to you before.

INTRODUCTION

I am a social worker, foster carer and social entrepreneur. I founded Bold Leap in 2020 and have since opened nine supported accommodation homes in England. I am currently in the process of opening my first children's residential home.

I will share the story of my journey, which began in Uganda. At the age of sixteen, I suffered the loss of my mother, uncle and grandparents. This devastation led me to a crisis point as I navigated life in the UK without parents and battled with suicide. Fortunately, I found refuge in Christianity, which led me to believe that I was not alone, that God was with me. The impossible became possible for me as I pursued the art of a purpose-driven life.

I started my career as a residential child worker. After I obtained a degree in social work from Birmingham City University in 2011, I worked for dozens of local authorities. One of the many highlights as a social worker was at the London Borough of Hammersmith and Fulham (LBHF). I was given the opportunity by Sara Scholey, the Head of Service for Children in Care and Care Leavers at that time. Sara was incredible as a leader and even more so as a person. She believed in my ability as a social worker and that confidence enabled me to perform to the best of my capability. I spent almost three years at LBHF. I went on to become a foster carer and then opened my own supported accommodation homes. Excitingly, I am now embarking on creating my own children's residential homes, which will bring me full circle.

Social Work and Beyond is a distillation of my knowledge and experience and will, therefore, appeal to those starting a career in social work as well as those considering an alternative path. The tools, tips and learning are the same, irrespective of your situation. I will share the lessons I have learned and equip you with strategies that you can apply in your practice and that will enable you to survive and thrive within social work.

As well as challenging and inspiring you to think about your purpose, I want more social workers to open their own businesses within social care. It is imperative that decisions are made in the interest of children rather than in the interest of profit, but there is a major issue with raising the necessary capital and managing finances. This was certainly my biggest challenge – one that made me pause and self-reflect, and one that I will help you to overcome.

INTRODUCTION

I will also explore various alternatives to social work. No, I am not advocating for you to leave the profession, because the profession needs you. What I am saying is that your skills as a social worker are transferable, so your current position need not be the end for you. There are many things in *Social Work and Beyond* that you may already know through your own experience as a social worker, but I feel that it is important to reinforce these very things to convince you that your skills are transferable – whether to other sectors or within the social care industry.

When I was just starting out as an inexperienced and newly qualified social worker, I didn't have a book or a guide to share stories and strategies that would have been very helpful to me at the start of my career. It is true that you cannot buy experience, but it is certainly helpful to know that others have walked the path you are setting out on, met the challenges you are facing and felt the pain you are suffering.

Having *Social Work and Beyond* to hand when you feel yourself overwhelmed by your workload and succumbing to burnout will quickly get you back on track and heading towards the life you know you want and, of course, deserve.

It takes courage to acknowledge that you need support – and even more to do something about getting it. *Social Work and Beyond* may be the first step in that direction, a direction that could change everything – the first step along the path that will light you up and bring you both success and satisfaction.

PART ONE
CHALLENGES

A career in social work can be highly rewarding, but it can also be severely challenging. Excessive workloads, high stress levels and low morale are rife among social workers, who are often at breaking point. Social workers' skills and interventions keep people safe from harm and change lives. But there simply aren't enough of them to deal with the increasing demand for their services.

In this first part of the book, I will look at the realities of social work today and the challenges that it poses. I will then look at the skills required to manage those challenges and suggest ways in which those skills can be honed and developed, not only to make your social work career less stressful and more satisfying, but also to allow you to transfer your skills to other areas (which we will be looking at in Part Two).

ONE
Meeting The Demands

The third Tuesday of March is World Social Work Day, an annual event organised by the International Federation of Social Workers. Its aim is to celebrate the achievements of social work, raise the visibility of social services for the future of societies and to defend social justice and human rights around the world. Social work is a worldwide profession because the challenges it faces are global challenges.

They include inadequate housing, substance abuse, mental health issues, domestic violence, economic deprivation, neglect, self-harm... The list goes on. These challenges are on the increase thanks to population growth, urbanisation, inflation, climate change, technological 'progress', rising divorce rates and the recent COVID pandemic. In the UK, there has been a significant rise in the number of children suffering mental health problems or not going to school and, consequently, coming into the care of local authorities because of the pandemic and the many social problems it has caused.

In the front line of defence against these challenges are social workers – the 'paramedics' of social ills who struggle daily to contain, control and remedy them. To empower individuals, families and communities to work through them. To navigate through the turmoil and overcome the obstacles they encounter so they then can become strong enough to 'carry their own cross' as it were. A social worker's aim is to shift communities and society away from suffering and unhappiness towards a brighter, safer, more fulfilling future.

Much of our work is, therefore, with children, since they are the future. Children are the primary victims of these social challenges, since they are a product of their environment in which they have little autonomy or agency. They suffer directly from poor parenting, a negative environment or culture and the effects of financial and mental health difficulties. If we can intervene early and influence the next generation, we can prevent these problems from being perpetuated down the generations.

The environment in which such children are being cared for, however, is changing. Where residential care homes were once run by former social workers with years of frontline expertise and a commitment to providing the best possible care, we are seeing them increasingly taken over by bosses with business experience, whose primary concern is to make profits and dividends for shareholders. It is a trend that is not only having potentially damaging consequences to those children and young people – and, ultimately, to our society – but also putting additional, and often extraneous, pressures on local authorities' budgets.

The nature of social work

If I were to be asked, 'What is social work?', I would say that it is about empowering other human beings, about creating a boldness within them to tackle the social challenges and problems that they encounter on a daily basis. The idea behind social work is not for children to be taken into care and kept there forever or for families to remain 'in the system' indefinitely. It is to socially empower these families to be able to stand on their own two feet.

This means that it begins with the individual. It starts with understanding how human beings think, how they behave, how they interact with each other and how they build relationships. On the one hand, it requires a knowledge of human biological and mental development, as well as of the societal issues and challenges humans face. On the other hand, it demands empathy, a caring nature, an appetite for social justice and the ability to develop relationships, as well as the belief and confidence that you can provide solutions and empower other human beings to improve their lives.

It is, therefore, essentially a practice-based profession. It does not – or should not – involve sitting on a chair and analysing data, but going out and delivering solutions to very real problems through one-to-one, family and small group services across a wide range of social issues. The practice is also evidence-based, which means more than simply recording everything that must be recorded so that it can be evidenced. A 2016 research paper by the Centre for Humanities Engaging Science, states that, in their daily practice,

> 'social workers may also draw on what they themselves have seen and heard, on their local knowledge, on theories, on observations that others, including family members, have reported to them and on the opinions of others. All of these become "evidence" when used to support a conclusion.'[1]

This, as we will see, is vitally important when it comes to accountability. The crucial and essential nature of social work means that it is highly regulated in England. All social workers in England are required to register annually (by 30th November) with Social Work England, which is a specialist body taking a new approach to regulating social workers in their vital roles. Social Work England believes in the power of collaboration and shares a common goal with those it regulates: to protect the public, enable positive change and, ultimately, improve people's lives. The same applies in other parts of the UK, where social workers are regulated by Social Care Wales, the Scottish Social Services Council and the Social Care Council of Northern Ireland.

Social workers can also become members of the British Association of Social Workers (BASW), a professional body that offers a variety of products and services, including training and advocacy training. As a BASW member, you are required to meet its standards of practice and abide by its code of ethics.

There are, of course, different elements to social work: different areas and departments you can work within and different types of service you can provide. Early Help is essentially the 'front door' service within social work, dealing with initial enquiries and referrals which are aimed at improving outcomes for children or preventing the escalation of need or risk.

Child in Need looks at referrals that have been 'flagged' as causing concern. In these cases, the local authority will see whether the child can be supported in their own home. A Child in Need plan will be drafted and periodically reviewed to see how effectively the risks are being managed. If the plan isn't working, the local authority will implement a Child Protection Plan. If that also fails, they will apply to a court to share parental responsibility for the child. When a child is looked after by the local authority, there are six-monthly reviews (LAC reviews), which impose long lists of tasks on social workers.

Whatever the approach adopted and the level of intervention required, social workers predominantly work with families to find solutions to both social and personal challenges. Their ultimate responsibility is to safeguard every child that is self-referred or referred by agencies to the local authority. This means that they must collaborate with a number of other agencies, including the police and representatives of the health sector and the education sector.

Multi-agency collaboration

The police have a very important part to play in addressing social issues. For example, if a mother or father or a couple are in a domestic dispute and there are children in the home, the police have a duty of care towards the child (or children) and must safeguard them against violence, abuse, neglect or mistreatment if necessary (ie, if they feel the children to be at risk) by taking them into police protection. Police officers often take part in important meetings with social workers, particularly around sexual exploitation and child safety, as well as youth crime.

Since virtually all children over the age of three are in education, schools also have a critical role to play in their safeguarding. If there is a concern within a school setting that a child is suffering abuse or neglect – for example, if they come to school with unexplained bruising – they must refer the case to social services.

And, of course, there is interaction between social workers and health workers, including GPs, nurses and midwives. Just as a teacher or school might report potential neglect or abuse, so GPs should refer suspicious cases to the local authority. Sadly, this doesn't always happen, and we have all seen inquests and inquiries into baby and child deaths where the signs are not picked up or flagged, with tragic consequences. Oddly, the health sector and other professions often escape criticism in such cases, while social workers take the brunt of the blame.

If a child or young person is being looked after by the local authority, they must have a health assessment every six or twelve months, which requires collaboration with nursing staff. In cases where a decision is made by the courts for an unborn child to be removed from their mother at birth, the social worker will have to interact with the midwife to manage what can be a very painful experience. Social workers must also interact with psychotherapists through a 'branch' of the NHS called Child and Adolescent Mental Health Services (CAMHS),* which is responsible for treating young people with emotional, behavioural or mental health difficulties and those suffering from trauma.

Multi-agency collaboration is not a new practice. As early as the mid-nineteenth century, health and social services were working hard to reduce poverty in England. But it was not until the 1980s, during the Thatcher government, that the foundations of multi-agency partnership working were laid. Practitioners from many agencies now shared their goals, tasks and responsibilities, allowing them to evaluate an individual's issues from multiple perspectives rather than focusing on a specific area. Multi-agency working has since spread across the whole system of help, support and

---

* You might also see CYPMHS, which stands for 'Children and Young People's Mental Health Services'.

protection for children and their families, with the aim of adopting a child-centred approach while maintaining a whole-family focus.

However, it is the social worker who must 'steer the ship', coordinate the relevant action plan and take ultimate responsibility for safeguarding. When a child is under a Child Protection Plan, for example, social workers and other agents regularly meet the child and their parents to ensure that the plan is working safely and effectively.

The government constantly strives to regulate and facilitate such collaboration through legislation and statutory guidance such as 'Working Together to Safeguard Children' (1999, revised in 2006, 2013, 2015, 2018 and 2023)[2] but as we know, there are often 'gaps' in this collaboration and tragedies that might have been prevented by closer or more effective interaction occur every year.

So, social work is not just about social workers. We all have a moral obligation to do the right thing when it comes to the safety and welfare of children in our society. If we have a concern or are aware of something happening in our vicinity, we must act – not necessarily physically, but by speaking up about it – because this could make the difference between life and death. To use the old African proverb, 'It takes a village to raise a child.' In other words, safeguarding is a community job description, and we are all accountable.

Nevertheless, the onus falls heavily on social workers, who are coming under increasing pressure from all sides to deliver results. I want to look at these pressures before going on to discuss some possible ways of dealing with them.

Challenges

As we have seen, one of the biggest challenges facing social workers today is working effectively and coherently with other agencies. This requires a high level of understanding, diplomacy and negotiating skills, since it is essential for the various parties to be 'on the same team', as opposed to pursuing separate and potentially conflicting agendas.

Social work often involves following a plan: there are Child Protection Plans, Pathway Plans, Care Plans... All these need to be carried out in conjunction with several other parties, including, as we have said, the police, education and health authorities, but also parents and children themselves. It is essential, but not always easy, to get the views of children involved in any Plan. The reason there are inquests and reports into child deaths, for example, is often that insufficient attention has been paid to the children's or the parents' views or that the various agencies involved in their safeguarding aren't working effectively enough together.

It is also symptomatic of an increasing 'culture of blame', where someone must be found responsible for every mishap. Again, as we have seen, the 'blame' all too often falls on social workers, who are seen to have 'failed' in their duties and responsibilities. This results in a government 'blame culture' and negative narratives around social work that has tirelessly worked to deliver support, compassion and kindness to children and families hand in hand with undertaking assessments and safeguarding investigations in challenging circumstances. Disappointingly, this leads to a burden of expectation that can be hard to bear.

Another challenge is the sheer workload social workers must contend with due to the simple fact that there are not enough social workers in England and elsewhere. In recent years, numbers have diminished, while the population and society's problems and issues have increased.

Asking social workers today what their top three challenges are, I find that 99% of them complain of a high caseload. In my own experience, I might have twenty children to case manage at any one time. Inevitably, the greater the workload, the more the quality of work becomes diluted. Even working full-time, it is humanly impossible to meet all the deadlines, achieve the KPIs and deliver the required outcomes.

High workloads lead to a whole list of consequences among social workers, such as stress, anxiety and burnout, or a total inability to function (which we will be looking at in more detail in the following chapters). When you are dealing with people in need and in desperate situations, you really cannot afford not to be producing your A game.

As I have mentioned, social work is a practice-based profession. Another challenge is that social work qualifications such as degrees don't necessarily prepare you adequately for the reality of such a fast-paced, hands-on role. The policies and theories and strategies and models you are told to embrace and absorb don't always apply. The lecture room and the classroom don't really teach you to be relational or social or to understand another person's social challenges. These are things you must learn on the job, because human beings aren't like textbooks, which is tough.

As a social worker you need to be something of a chameleon. Sometimes you will need to be a 'teacher', providing information. Sometimes a 'solicitor', explaining the law. Sometimes a counsellor, giving advice. Sometimes you will need to be empathetic, simply lending an understanding ear and sometimes you will need to be dogmatic and stern, setting boundaries and issuing instructions. On most days, you will need to be all those things, changing your approach from moment to moment. It can be demanding. It can be exhausting.

You will need to be flexible in other ways, too, given that you are operating in a constantly shifting environment. Policies and practices will change and evolve and, with them, your responsibilities and the expectations others have of you.

I remember feeling that I had to 'sink or swim' when I started my first job and was literally struggling to catch my breath. The demand was high, the expectations were high, and, somehow, I had to find my place in a very turbulent environment. Which brings us to the question: Do you have the resilience, the boldness and the confidence that it takes not to sink, not be overwhelmed, but to survive and thrive? This is a question we will be trying to answer in the following chapters.

Accountability

In 2019, Social Work England, the professional governing body for social workers in England, published a set of professional standards consisting of fifteen points that social workers are expected to adhere to. These can be found in full on their website: www.socialworkengland.org.uk.[3]

A few examples include working within legal and ethical frameworks and using their professional authority and judgement appropriately; using information from a range of appropriate sources to inform their assessments, to analyse risk and make professional decisions;

recognising where there may be bias in decision-making and addressing issues that arise from ethical dilemmas, conflicting information, or differing professional decisions and maintaining accurate, legible and up-to-date records documenting how decisions are reached.

Similar standards apply in other parts of the UK. One of the key principles outlined by BASW is that social workers should be prepared to account for and justify their judgements and actions to people who use their services, to employers and to the public, in terms that are comprehensible to the people concerned.[4]

We see from this that being transparent and professionally accountable is fundamental within social work – not surprisingly, considering that we are engaging with people to address major life challenges and the decisions we make can literally save lives (or not). This, however, puts a heavy burden of expectation on social workers, who are often made to feel that they must achieve perfection in everything they do – whether case loading or case managing or being responsible for others.

In the example I gave earlier of a referral being issued by a school for a child having unexplained bruising, a social worker will be sent to visit the child's home. If that social worker fails to cross their t's and dot their i's by asking all the right questions and being vigilant and fully aware of all the signs and markers and the child returns home to an environment in which there is serious domestic abuse, the social worker will need to account for their failure to safeguard and protect that child. It also means that many social workers live in fear of being blamed and labelled by an inquiry or inquest, as well as having to live with the resulting 'guilt'.

There is, or should be, another side to accountability, which is accepting when you are wrong or have made a bad call. This is something that needs to be addressed and encouraged within the industry, but that is another discussion.

Roles and responsibilities

The role of the social worker is changing. Like so many jobs in today's world, social work is becoming increasingly data driven. More and more time is spent on assessments and 'number-crunching', so that less and less time is available for meaningful work on the ground, on the frontline in schools and communities.

Add to this the constant cuts to budgets by local authorities and the result is, again, the overburdening of social workers and a lack of practitioners in the field. This impacts on the quality of their work with the service users. Speaking to social workers, I find this lack of resources one of the principal causes of dissatisfaction and stress factors we will be looking at in the following chapters.

Years ago, there were social work assistants who were not qualified, but helped social work teams to do some of the direct work on the ground. They were increasingly asked to undertake tasks that were beyond their skills and knowledge, with the result that social work assistants and others working in social work support roles such as community care workers became undervalued, underpaid and undertrained. Unfortunately, those positions have been significantly reduced, which only exacerbates the problem.

Lack of resources also means that there aren't enough skillsets in social work teams to be able to manage some of the more complex scenarios. There may, for example, be a shortage of family support workers, which puts pressure on the other members of the team to act as family support workers or to become therapists or counsellors. Equally, in social work there is not always sufficient time to complete all relevant and required tasks – such that time itself can become the greatest enemy.

All the above factors are a major deterrent to people entering the profession, as well as a major cause of people leaving the profession. There are, as we shall see in Chapter 4, several options for career progression within social work, but many look to transfer their skills to other sectors. We will be looking at those transferable skills in the next chapter.

Of course, you must prove yourself within the profession before you will be able to develop your career either within it or elsewhere. You cannot buy experience. You must gain it. It will change you and add value to you. It will complete you as a person. It took me ten years to 'earn my stripes', as my story illustrates.

My story

I was born in Uganda in the eighties. My father was from a political background and he came to the UK in the late eighties to study. He achieved a Master of Arts in Developmental Administration and then a PhD in the same field at Birmingham University. We followed him as a family, and I spent the next twelve years here. We returned to Uganda because my dad wanted to resume his career in politics. I was sixteen. That's when I had my first encounter with tragedy and trauma. My mum died in a car crash.

I spent a year in Uganda, but I wasn't comfortable there, so I came back to the UK when I was seventeen and then had to rebuild my life. I completed my GCSEs and A-levels. My mum was a very caring individual and had spent her career within social care. I was inspired by her, so social work was the natural field for me to go into.

My social work journey began as a residential child support worker in several children's homes throughout England. I then embarked on a three-year social work degree at Birmingham City University. During that period, I spent six months working as a Young Persons' Advisor for Shaftesbury Young People in Wolverhampton. After graduating in 2012, I spent eleven years working for a dozen different local authorities in England, as well as becoming a foster carer.

But during that time, I increasingly felt frustrated and burnt out. I needed more. I didn't have the right work/life balance. I wanted more autonomy and control, more authority, more flexibility and more money. I knew I could do more. But which way should I turn? What was the alternative?

I'd always had a desire for entrepreneurship, for getting into business. So, I thought, 'How do I use my social work skills and transfer those into the business world?' My journey to entrepreneurship was not a smooth one. First, in 2017, I set up a supported accommodation company with another social worker. When that didn't work out because we had different output and work ethics, I started a second one with a close friend. Finally, after two years of getting nowhere, I set up on my own as CLA Placements. In 2020, I changed the company name to Bold Leap – an organisation dedicated to providing care, support and accommodation for children in care. Eventually, in March 2023, I was able to stop practising as a social worker and became a full-time operations director at Bold Leap. During this period, I began the process of registering Bold Leap as a supported accommodation service and children's home with Ofsted. The process was testing, and I learned the art of being a conscious social work entrepreneur. Interestingly, I returned to social work practice in August 2024 and the break was refreshing. Importantly, I feel the advantage to remaining within the social work profession is that it has kept me grounded to the mission at hand: creating opportunities for children in care to excel.

Our objective is to work with local authorities to ensure that these children and young people have a platform to succeed in life. It's a fascinating sector, because when a child comes into care, the local authority becomes the Corporate Parent. Put simply, the term 'Corporate Parent' means that the council, elected members, employees and partner agencies have collective responsibility for providing the best possible care and safeguarding for the children who are looked after by them.

As I write this, I am in the process of opening my first children's home. In a sense, I have come full circle from being a support worker in a children's home to owning and running my own home.

Summary

Social work is a vital and valuable profession, recognised and celebrated throughout the world. It aims to tackle global challenges such as deprivation, neglect and abuse, particularly against children. Social workers are the 'paramedics' of social ills, who struggle daily to shift communities towards a happier and safer future by safeguarding and empowering children and young people to stand on their own two feet.

This work is itself highly challenging, requiring not only knowledge, understanding and empathy, but also adherence to strict regulations and procedures. The ability to collaborate and negotiate with other agencies and the capacity to cope with a high workload can have adverse consequences at both a professional and a personal level.

Social workers have great responsibility and are accountable for their decisions and actions, since 'the buck stops with them'. Their roles are constantly changing, generally moving away from hands-on practice towards reporting and number-crunching, and both resources and support are often scarce.

All this requires the development of a variety of skills, which we will look at in the next chapter.

TWO
Honing Your Skills

We have looked at some of the challenges of being a social worker today. In this chapter I will look at how to manage these challenges and become effective and efficient as a social worker.

As we have seen, a variety of skills are essential to the role of a social worker. As well as needing to be personable and relatable and have good interpersonal skills, you must be able to work under pressure and meet deadlines. You must be able to co-operate and collaborate with other agencies and you must not allow the demands of your work to get on top of you.

SOCIAL WORK AND BEYOND

To do all this effectively and efficiently, you must be well organised and plan your work meticulously, you must hone your communication skills and you must develop resilience. I will suggest ways in which you can achieve these things.

Most importantly, in the context of this book, I will show that all these skillsets are transferable and can be utilised in other sectors of social work and in other industries. For example, being a frontline social worker equips you to deal with problems and crises, both foreseen and unforeseen. This is an invaluable skill which is transferable to any and every other area of work.

Another essential part of your day-to-day work is achieving outcomes and evidencing that those outcomes are being achieved. This is second nature to you, so you may not realise what an important (and transferable) skill it is.

As I have said, however, before branching out into other areas, you will need to survive and thrive within social work. To learn as much as you can, because it will change you. It will add value to you. It will complete you as a person.

Organisation and planning

Organisational skills are a key part of a social worker's 'toolbox'. Hand in hand with these is the ability to plan effectively. As the old saying goes, 'If you fail to plan, you plan to fail,' – and in the world of social work, poor planning can cost lives.

The world of social work can be hectic and challenging in many respects, with a high volume of caseloads and literally not enough hours in the day to do everything that needs to be done. You must often make your own decisions as to what to do and when; you cannot simply rely on a line manager to do this for you, but must think on your feet. Managing your time effectively is essential.

After years of 'learning the hard way' (and making many mistakes), I would like to share some tips on how to be organised from my own experience.

1. Keep a calendar or a diary

Keep a calendar or a diary so that not only you but, crucially, others know where you are going to be throughout the week. Make sure it is always up to date and that you book in all your appointments, meetings and visits, as well as time for admin.

One of the managers I worked with early in my career once said to me, 'Peter, allocate one day a week for admin.' I didn't really understand. Why would I do that when there were so many more pressing demands on my time? In fact, I soon discovered that it makes a lot of sense, because if you are too busy running around doing fieldwork without leaving enough time for the admin, you will always be playing catchup. Setting aside one day a week purely for administration will help you to manage your workload more effectively.

As I have just mentioned, a key benefit of keeping a calendar is that your colleagues, manager and everyone else that you work with knows what you are doing and where you are at any time on any day. This not only saves them time not having to 'chase' you but it also has safety implications. If you are ever not where you should be, others will know to check that you are safe and well.

2. Always carry a notepad

When you visit homes or schools, whether you are meeting a young person or a family, a teacher or safeguarding officer, a doctor or nurse, always make a record of your conversations. This will ensure that when it comes to doing the data entry afterwards, you won't need to remember everything that was said and discussed as you will have the notes with you.

A frequent critique of social workers is that when a child turns eighteen and they read through their files (which can be a traumatic enough experience), they find errors that can affect their self-image and confidence, as well as their faith in the social work profession. Keeping detailed notes also helps with accountability in that you can check exactly what has happened and what actions you have taken in a particular case. As we have seen, social work is evidence-based and 'if it wasn't recorded, it didn't happen.' When it comes to court proceedings (and these can sometimes go on for six months or more), having complete, accurate and factual notes can save a lot of time, misunderstandings and even miscarriages of justice.

3. Have a weekly routine

Having a weekly routine is another way to stay organised. I have suggested spending one day a week doing admin. If you can, make this the same day each week and allocate other regular tasks to particular days so that you always know what you are doing today, tomorrow and next week.

Organising your workspace when you are in the office (or at home if you are hybrid working) is equally important. It shows that you are rigorous in your work, it saves you time and it reduces the likelihood of succumbing to stress and anxiety.

4. Know 'where you are' with each case

You should always know 'where you are' with each case in terms of the plan that is being followed and be able to answer questions such as:

- Where are we going with this one?
- What's the direction for this child?
- What's happening in the next six months?
- What's the plan for the next twelve months?

5. Make the most efficient use of your time

You also need to know where you are in a purely physical sense. By that, I mean organising your meetings and visits to make the most efficient use of your time. If, for example, you need to see several children and they are all in the same area, try to arrange to see them all in one day. This will save you travelling time. Even if it is only half an hour here and an hour there, you will soon notice the benefit of good planning.

Different people manage their time in different ways, and there is no 'one size fits all' solution. Some people value to-do lists, for example, while others avoid them like the plague on the basis that they always seem to get longer.

6. Learn the timeboxing technique

Another system many social workers (and other busy people) swear by is known as 'timeboxing'. There are various versions of this method, for example, the Pomodoro® Technique, developed by Francesco Cirillo in the late 1980s.[5] The process involves allocating a fixed or limited time to specific activities or tasks. Not all jobs are equally important, so give priority to the most critical tasks by allocating them to your most productive hours.

In rather the same way as you might work through an exam, once the allotted time ends, you move on to your next task. Timeboxing can give your working day a more structured feel, keep you focused on each task and make it seem more manageable, reduce your sense of overwhelm, and, above all, put you in control of your work rather than letting it control you. It will also enable you to ensure that you have regular breaks.

When working out how much time to allow for each type of activity, whether meetings, admin, research or phone calls, overestimate rather than underestimating, allowing for the inevitable problems, emergencies and interruptions. Use a timer or alarm to keep you on track and keep a record of how you performed. At the end of each week, review your timeboxes and adjust them if necessary to further improve your efficiency.

In the unpredictable world of social work, you will, of course, need to remain flexible and adjust your plan if necessary. Don't be discouraged if your timeboxes are initially hard to keep to. Like any new regime, timeboxing might at first seem restricting, but if you persist with it, you should soon start to feel the benefits.

Whatever system works for you, however, try not to confuse what is urgent with what is important and don't fall into the trap of crisis intervention or 'firefighting' – ie, simply reacting to each problem as and when it arises, regardless of its severity. In this connection, you might find the classic Eisenhower Matrix useful. Developed by Dwight D Eisenhower, this is a decision-making and time management tool to help effectively prioritise tasks according to their urgency and importance.[6]

Experience, of course, will help you to prioritise to recognise the cases and situations that require your urgent attention. This is not something you will learn 'in the abstract' as a student, or even in your early years of practice. It takes time. Experience will also teach you when you need to ask your colleagues to assist you or seek management oversight. Always remember there is only one you and, despite your best intentions, you cannot be everywhere at once.

7. Communicate more

It may seem paradoxical, but you can also save time by communicating more, rather than less. If you ignore voicemails and emails until you are ready and able to respond, you are likely to be 'chased', which will only create more messages to deal with. If, on the other hand, you reply immediately with a 'holding' message such as, 'Hi, thanks for your message. I'll get back to you within 24/72 hours,' (in the case of emails, this can be simply copied and pasted), you will buy yourself time to plan your answer.

This will also let parents, professionals and stakeholders know that you are prioritising them and carrying out due diligence rather than sending them an off-the-cuff response. Don't be afraid to be honest. If you don't know the answer to their question, send them a different holding message, for example, 'I don't have that information right now, but give me another couple of days and I'll get back to you.'

Good organisation doesn't happen overnight. It comes with effort and months and months of getting it right, making mistakes, getting it right again, making more mistakes and learning from those mistakes.

Communication

Like good organisation and planning, good communication is a vital skill to develop in all aspects of social work. You are dealing and working with people that are often sensitive and vulnerable and facing significant challenges, so communicating your intentions clearly is essential. One of the main criticisms of social workers is that they don't communicate effectively: they say one thing, but do another. It is important to be honest about your role, your intentions, the current situation, the objective and how you are going to get from A to B. Here are some tips on communication gained from my own experience.

1. You can never communicate too much

I once had a complaint against me because a father felt that I wasn't communicating enough. I wasn't keeping him fully updated on his child's case. From that, I learned that you can never do too much communicating. Make sure that whenever anything significant occurs that is relevant to a case, you update everyone concerned as soon as possible.

This is particularly important when multiple agencies are involved in a case. For example,

West Midlands Police might be dealing with a child in Birmingham, who then moves to London, requiring the Met Police and the relevant local authority in London to be updated on the case.

How and when you communicate is also significant: start as you mean to go on. When you are first allocated to a case or to a child, you should always make an introductory telephone call, so that the parents or school know that their case is being dealt with and have a real person to contact in connection with it. It sets the tone and reassures them that you are organised and competent.

Listening is a key part of communication that is often overlooked. As social workers we often find ourselves doing most of the talking and directing those whose safety we are responsible for. It is also vital to step back and listen to what the other person, the child or parent is saying and take stock of this.

2. 'Active' listening is a key part of communication

'Active' listening requires total concentration so that you hear, understand and remember what the other person says. It also means showing the speaker that you are listening and understanding through both non-verbal and verbal responses. The former include nodding, smiling and taking notes; the latter include 'echoing' what the speaker says and giving feedback, which will reduce the chance of misunderstanding.

Try not to interrupt. Let the speaker finish before responding. If you need more information, ask open rather than closed questions. For example, 'How did you feel?' is preferable to, 'Did you feel bad?' Above all, avoid expressing personal opinions or judgements; your job is to understand, not to agree or disagree.

Active listening not only makes you more effective and efficient by not having to ask for things to be repeated or missing vital details and by enabling you to pick up unspoken signals; it also builds trust in the people you are dealing with, which is obviously essential in situations where they are sharing highly personal, sensitive and often painful information.

To make active listening possible, you must avoid and prevent all distractions, particularly noise and the likelihood of being interrupted (eg, by ringing phones). Make sure that you are in a quiet place and that all mobiles are switched off before you begin any discussion or meeting.

3. Evidence and record meetings

Once again, evidencing and recording meetings and conversations is critical whether it is a phone call to a solicitor or barrister, a conversation with a teacher or a meeting with parents or children. You never know when that evidence might be needed in the future – perhaps at a child protection conference or even in court proceedings.

Always take down the name and contact details of fellow professionals who attend meetings with you (and make a note of any who should be attending, but aren't) so that you can contact them directly afterwards. Similarly, you should always share your contact information so that they can easily get in touch with you if they need to. Always request the minutes of the meeting so that you can refer to what was discussed and the action points that were agreed upon.

You should also always be sure to follow up meetings and conversations with a written communication of some kind, whether a letter, an email or even a text or WhatsApp message. This will prevent any doubt or uncertainty as to what was discussed and agreed.

4. Be open with your colleagues

Just as you should be open and honest with those whose cases you are dealing with, you should also be upfront with your colleagues and managers. If you are having a bad day or struggling to cope with your workload, tell them. Not only might they be able to help, but you will also reduce any potential knock-on effects that you not performing at your best might have on them.

Most importantly, if you are moving on to another department or handing over a case to a colleague, make sure that everyone who needs to be in the know does so that there are no 'gaps' in communication.

The more we communicate effectively, the better chance we have of dealing with the risks facing young people and adults and the social problems and challenges that we face within social work. Always remember that you are working with families and children, not against them, and one of the things that will work most damagingly against them is lack of communication.

Resilience

The many challenges inherent in a career in social work mean that it commands the practitioner (ie, you) to have considerable mental and emotional resilience. In my experience, this is perhaps the single most important quality for you to build on and strengthen. And it is a 'skill' that you need to constantly work on, because the more resilient you are, the better you will be able to manage the demands of the job and the longer you will be able to stay in the industry.

Resilience is like a shield that will protect your wellbeing, and developing resilience is, in fact, more an art than a skill. A mental and emotional martial art, if you like. You need to find and use your inner strength to defend yourself against the negative emotional impact of some horrific cases you will have to deal with, as well as the constant pressure that comes with the job, which can not only affect the quality of your work but also lead to stress, anxiety and burnout. Here are some further tips on how to develop and maintain resilience.

1. Don't get emotionally involved

The first thing I always tell social workers is, 'Don't get emotionally involved in the cases you deal with.' If you become engrossed or entangled in a case, this will have an impact on your ability to manage it effectively. It is, therefore, essential to constantly 'step back' and reflect on the case to see clearly how it needs to be dealt with. Yes, you must be supportive, but this requires you to be resilient, because the children and families you are working with are in a highly challenging situation themselves and will be looking to you to be strong in the face of adversity.

This, of course, is easier said than done. But, like charity, resilience begins 'at home'. This means that you must build your own support network among your colleagues as well as your family and friends. Don't be afraid to 'offload' and share your concerns with others. Take them aside and bounce ideas off them. Use your monthly supervisions with your team manager, for example, to reflect and regroup. Often simply talking things through helps to bring them into focus.

All this will be easier if you are fortunate enough to be working under a good manager. But be aware that managers are under pressure, too, and may not have the time or the expertise to give you the help and support you might need. It is therefore largely up to you to self-manage, as explained in this chapter.

Make sure also that you associate with people who have a positive influence on you and that you exert a positive influence on them. There is strength in numbers, but only if the right people make up those numbers.

2. Don't try to be superhuman

Social workers often try to come across as indestructible, able to contend with any and every challenge that comes their way. No problem. Bring it on. But no one is superhuman. We all have our own personal challenges to deal with as well, our own inner turmoil of doubts and fears, and these must be constantly faced up to and dealt with.

This also means that it is essential to set clear boundaries between your work and your personal life. By that I mean, don't take your work home. The moment you start taking work home as a social worker is the moment you start to lose control of your life. This, too, is easy for me to say. Accountants can simply switch off at 5 o'clock and go home; the numbers can wait. When you are working with a family and there is a safeguarding crisis, it can seem almost criminal to 'leave it until tomorrow'. But a good work/life balance is fundamental to your effectiveness as a social worker. Taking a break will refresh and invigorate you so that you are even more effective when you pick up the case again the next day. There is an element of selfishness here, but always remember: you are no good to a child in need of care if you aren't caring for yourself.

3. Self-care is vital

Self-care is greatly underrated and, in fact, it is virtually ignored within social work. The focus is on achieving outcomes and solving problems – so much so that the social worker is often forgotten in the process. Our managers, who of course are themselves under great pressure, generally don't invest enough in our wellbeing, which means that it is even more important for you to regularly check in on it yourself.

Putting yourself first is very important. Look at your own needs and the signals your body is giving you: am I overtired? Stressed? Do I need some downtime? Don't ignore the signs and think you will 'be OK'.

By their very nature, social workers are selfless people, working not for money or status or fame, but for the betterment of other people. That inherent altruism means that we often fail to stand up for ourselves (or for our profession), but it is vital sometimes to put yourself first.

One of the things I learned over my years as a social worker is the importance of taking short breaks that increase your energy levels and make you more alert and more focused on the task at hand. Don't forfeit the leave you are entitled to. If you can't afford extended holidays, take a Friday off every month and treat yourself to a long weekend away or at home.

Being organised is another way to boost your resilience. Earlier in this chapter, we talked about the importance of good organisation and planning to increase your efficiency and effectiveness, but they are equally important in terms of maintaining your resilience. It is hard to feel resilient if you are constantly flustered and confused by a lack of organisation.

Outside of work, do things that you like doing, whether exercising, reading, cooking or simply spending time with friends or family – things that will strengthen you and refill your fuel tank.

4. Model resilience

Finally, it is vital for you to model resilience, not only to the families and children you are working with, but also to your colleagues – especially if you are managing others. This will inspire and motivate them and build a sense of collective resilience: 'He's been through it and come out strong, so I can too.'

Make sure that you are provided adequate supervision. I know from the social workers I speak to that supervision isn't happening enough, which means that there is no space for the social worker to reflect on practice and to offload about the emotional challenges and obstacles they are facing. It is, therefore, incumbent upon you as a manager to create a platform – a space for supervision where social workers can be open and honest about how they are feeling without being criticised or devalued; a 'team culture' of trust and support. This is another way of building emotional resilience.

Summary

To deal effectively with the many challenges of the job without succumbing to stress or burnout, social workers require a variety of skills. They must, of course, be good problem-solvers, but also efficient planners. They must be well organised (keeping a diary, setting aside time for administration, making detailed notes, establishing a work routine and 'timeboxing'), as well as flexible and able to adjust their priorities according to circumstances.

They must be good communicators, always keeping everyone 'in the loop' while not being afraid to be honest, as well as good listeners, cultivating the art of 'active' listening and always remembering to record conversations and contact information. They must also be both mentally and emotionally resilient in order not to be affected by the cases they deal with or let them 'spill over' into their private life.

The importance of self-care is often overlooked, especially by social workers themselves. Remember that you cannot look after others unless you first look after yourself.

THREE
Preparing Yourself

We have looked at some of the challenges faced by social workers today, at the skills needed for the job and how to sharpen these. But improving our day-to-day working life is often not enough to ensure that we thrive, or even survive, in our increasingly demanding environment.

The demands are now such that record numbers are leaving the profession every year. In 2022, a total of 5,400 social workers left the profession in 2022 – a 9% rise on the previous year, and the highest number since 2017.[7] Many suffer failed relationships or become alienated from their children because their work has taken over their entire lives. Social workers often end up on medication or in hospital with stress-related illnesses and a few go as far as taking their own lives because they see no way out of the cycle of constant pressure and overload.

In this chapter, I look at some of the things you can do outside your work environment to help you to cope with your role as a social worker and, ultimately, to prepare yourself – mind, body and spirit – for a career beyond social work.

Self-evaluation

Preparing yourself begins with a process of self-reflection and self-evaluation. Not only is this required as part of your registration as a social worker (as I will discuss below), but it is also an essential part of your development as a person. Self-evaluation is greatly underrated; it is massively important if you want to perform at the highest level.

It isn't something to be done reluctantly and hurriedly. Self-evaluation is something that should be done regularly throughout every

PREPARING YOURSELF

day. It enables you to review your experiences to help make positive changes for your future practice. It turns your experiences into learning and helps you improve your practice in a way that is right for you. 'Wait a minute,' I hear you say. 'I don't even have time to grab a coffee, let alone gaze at my navel!' Just as it's important to organise your work tasks to make the most efficient use of your time, so it is crucial to build some time into your schedule to 'work' on yourself.

Think of it like buying Christmas presents: do you want to have to rush around on Christmas Eve grabbing anything and everything that will 'do' as a gift, or would you rather buy them throughout the year whenever you see something that a particular person might like so that by the beginning of December you have already done all your Christmas shopping?

In an ideal world, self-evaluation will be part of your management supervision sessions, during which you can discuss and assess your decision-making, your practice, your performance, your KPIs and your emotional wellbeing with your team manager. But this doesn't always happen. Inadequate quality and frequency of supervision were found to have been a factor in two-thirds of the local reviews of serious cases in 2021 analysed by the Child Safeguarding Practice Review Panel for its annual report.[8] Against a backdrop of rapid societal changes, social workers must therefore increasingly look for their own innovative solutions to their work with clients. You are expected to spend your day looking after other people, but who is looking after you? If no one else is, then you must.

Self-evaluation is a skill like any other, which requires commitment, patience and practice to develop. Good social workers are constantly evaluating themselves, thinking, analysing and reflecting on everything they do, both at work and outside work. They do so both consciously and, after a while, subconsciously, in a sort of permanent feedback loop that informs every aspect of their lives.

Try to get into the habit, after carrying out any task, of asking yourself: 'How did that go? What went well, what didn't, and why? Could I have done better and, if so, how?' Make notes and keep a journal or diary of thoughts and actions so that you can see the areas you need to work on and, by referring back, how you are progressing.

Training

The lessons you take from your self-evaluation will enable you to clearly see the areas you need to improve on, which leads us on to training. Again, you may be thinking, 'My workload is so intense, I don't have time for training.' But, as you know, continual professional development (CPD) is a requirement for registration as a social worker, and every 30th November you must produce evidence that you are continually developing your practice. In doing so, you demonstrate to the public that you continue to be fit to practise as a social worker.

Like self-evaluation, training should be provided by your employer, whether you are working for a local authority or in the private sector. Local authorities, for example, will specify mandatory training each year. This, however, tends to be around practice and competency, ie, around making sure that you remain up to date with legislation and best practice so that you do a good job. It might cover safeguarding or child sexual exploitation, missing persons policy, trauma therapy, or simply first aid. It may not be connected to the needs you have identified through your self-evaluation process.

Since it is ultimately up to you to undertake training, make sure you allow time for it. As with self-evaluation, you should include regular training periods in your work timetable so that you don't miss out or must cram all your required training into the month before registration.

Learning

Self-evaluation and training may ultimately be your own responsibility, but self-development also involves learning, which requires external input.

Hopefully, having trained to be a social worker, you will already love learning. You will at least have trained your mind to learn, since you have had to learn a lot to get where you are: about core skills for practice, law and safeguarding, theories and methods for social work practice, critical reflective practice and child development.

No matter how well trained or experienced you are, however, there is always something to learn. This can be done by reading, attending talks, seminars and conferences, or consulting a social work coach – which is something I will be recommending, especially if you are planning to start a business.

Unlike some other professions, social work offers virtually nothing in the way of mentoring schemes. There are, however, an increasing number of independent consultancy firms that offer mentoring programmes aimed at improving wellbeing and work/life balance and preventing burnout among social workers.

Once again, using such services involves a commitment of time, not to mention money, but, in my opinion, it is imperative if you want to perform to the highest level that you can and prepare yourself for other career opportunities.

Discipline

In the last chapter, we looked at resilience and how to develop it. Hand in hand with that goes discipline, which is another greatly underrated 'skill'. Discipline means knowing what your limits are as a social worker, knowing where your ceiling is, knowing when you are running out of fuel. Discipline means knowing when to say to yourself, 'This is my cutting-off point;

I'm done here. Otherwise, I'm not going to be effective towards the children, the families, my colleagues and stakeholders.'

Like so many things in the social worker's toolkit, discipline comes largely through experience, but it can also be acquired through learning.

Avoiding burnout

Burnout can occur when you experience long-term stress and is recognised by the World Health Organization (WHO) as an 'occupational phenomenon'. According to Mental Health UK, it is a 'state of physical and emotional exhaustion'. The organisation lists common signs of burnout, which include feeling tired, drained, overwhelmed or helpless. You may feel detached and cynical about life. It is also common to experience self-doubt, to blame yourself for poor performance or to procrastinate and take longer than usual to get things done.[9]

Burnout causes you to lose the ability to effectively meet the demands of your job, which can have knock-on effects on other areas of your life.

PREPARING YOURSELF

Burnout isn't something which will just go away if you 'work through it'. In fact, it can get worse and increasingly damage your mental and physical health unless you address the issues that are causing it. The factors identified by Mental Health UK as significantly contributing towards burnout include caring for others – in other words, for social workers it is literally an occupational hazard – and 'poor sleep' (which we will look at next), as well as worries about money and job security.[10]

According to a recent report by The British Psychological Society, 1.6 million days are lost each year to work stress and mental health issues in social care today.[11] More than three-quarters of the 114 local authorities in England identified 'burnout' as the biggest single cause of time off among social workers.

How can we avoid burnout? There are several steps that can reduce the likelihood of suffering from burnout:

- Drinking lots of water throughout the day.
- Taking regular breaks.
- Avoid staying in front of your screen for extended periods of time.

- Going for daily walks.
- Sleeping well (see below).

Sleep

Among the primary predictors of burnout is lack of sleep.[12] This is because chronic stress affects the biological processes that make you sleep. And, of course, it is a vicious circle because lack of sleep increases stress levels.[13]

Persistent lack of sleep (also known as sleep debt) can increase our reaction times, make us more sensitive to stress and even reduce our capacity for empathy – a critical factor for social workers.

Conversely, sleep enables your brain to 'process' the information it has been bombarded with during the day. How often do you wake up with the 'answer' to a problem that has been worrying you?

So, what can we do to keep our sleep debt to a minimum and reduce the risk of burnout? Here are a few useful strategies:

- Establish a consistent sleep schedule and aim for the same number of hours sleep every night.

- Extend your sleep period whenever possible, by either going to bed a little earlier in the evening or staying in bed a little longer in the morning. Don't, however, allow yourself to 'nap' in the evening, which can be detrimental to your night's sleep.

- Wind down before going to bed: avoid bright lights and exercise late in the evening and make sure you have 'got rid of' your worries before retiring. A hot bath is a good way of relaxing before bed.

- Avoid eating late in the evening and stop drinking caffeine or alcohol well before bedtime.

Achieving a work/life balance

To be organised in our work, however, we must first organise ourselves within our personal lives. It is simply not possible to incorporate an organised work routine into a chaotic lifestyle.

Equally, if we don't take care of ourselves first, then we can't effectively help someone else. If we can't make sure as social workers that we are leading a healthy and balanced life, then we aren't going to be able to sustain the rhythm we need to best serve the children and families that we work with and support.

Having a 'work/life balance' is not just about not letting work take over your life; it is also about not letting life invade and disrupt your work. Routine is a vital part of both work and life. So, it is important to start by assessing your personal life and making sure that it is well organised. Then you can apply the same principles to your work life.

Admittedly, it can be difficult at times to keep work and the rest of your life separate. Social work is such an emotional and emotive profession that it can be particularly hard to 'switch off' at 5 o'clock, but it is very important to do so. This requires discipline, as we discussed earlier, and practice. If you are struggling to find a work/life balance, consider the following tips:

- Self-reflect: Practise self-reflection often so that you can recognise whether you are in balance or not before it is too late.

- Set attainable goals every day: The daily tasks as a social worker will likely vary according to your clients' situation. Write down a list of priorities and check each task off throughout the day. This can help you feel a sense of control and accomplishment when things get hectic. Remember to be realistic with goals and deadlines.

- Take a break: It might not seem like you have fifteen minutes to spare some days, but there is always time to take a break. Walking away from work can help clear your mind and improve your ability to handle tasks and make better decisions when you return to work.

- Make time for yourself: You take your job very seriously, but that doesn't mean it should define you. Making time for yourself improves mental health and overall satisfaction with life. Whether you enjoy taking a stroll in the park, exercising with friends or treating yourself to a spa day, it's critical to prioritise 'me time'.

- Ask for flexibility: If your workload has become unbearable, don't be afraid to ask your employer for flexibility. Time off can give you the mental clarity you need to properly assist and care for your clients in the future.

- Reach out for support: Social workers need support as much as anyone else, but the challenging nature of the job might require you to expand your social support network. Meeting a colleague over coffee or tea to let off steam, reconnect or prepare yourself for a particularly busy period can provide some stress relief, as can catching up with friends and family.

Finding your why

The final stage in preparing yourself for a wider career consists in reflecting and looking within yourself, as you did in the self-evaluation stage, to find your purpose – not only in your career, but also in life. This is what I like to call 'finding your why'.

Purpose is an essential element of you. It is the reason you are on the planet at this time in history. Your very existence is wrapped up in the things you are here to fulfil. The struggles along the way are only meant to shape you for your purpose.

PREPARING YOURSELF

This is no simple task because you might have found who you are as a social worker by now, but as a practitioner, you may seem to have lost sight of who you are as a person (your identity) and of your vision and purpose.

It's time to remind yourself of why you wanted to become a social worker: of the type of person you are, of your attributes and skills. Was it because you wanted to be the voice for the voiceless, to advocate for those who are incapable of advocating, to impact the lives of the disadvantaged and the marginalised and the vulnerable and the incapable? In sum, to be an agent of change for the greater good? I would be surprised if it wasn't, since these are the reasons given by most Year 1 students when asked why they have enrolled on a social work course.

These are the things you want to do; *this* is your why – not filling in forms and completing progress reports and undergoing assessments.

Think also about the lessons you have learned about life, look at your other interests, open your horizons and see what other directions you might head in. In Part Two of this book, we will look at some of those, but first you must be able to take the leap and you must have belief in yourself.

It is also important not to feel guilty if you are thinking of exiting the profession; not to feel that you are 'quitting' or giving up or failing. It is about looking in the mirror and saying, 'I've given everything I have to this, and now it's time to take a leap in a different direction.'

Case studies

I have spoken to many social workers about the challenges they face, how they deal with them, and what advice they would give to those starting out in the profession. I would like to share (with their permission) some of their insights here.*

MIKE

'I qualified as a social worker in 2011 and have worked in the areas of Children in Care, Child Protection and Assessment. For me, the major challenges presented by the work are the high caseloads, the volume of (repetitive)

---

* Both names have been changed.

paperwork, a lack of resources and bullying by management. The majority of families need a therapy approach, as they are dealing with a lot of trauma. I want to do the deep and direct work with them, but so much of what I must do is surface level (ticking boxes). I have raised these issues but nothing changes; so, now I just focus on what I can do.

'Something I see all too often is parents who have been in care themselves in their teens or at a very young age having their own children removed. There is a massive failure in the system that leads to a repeated cycle of care. The government has caused so much damage to the system that it isn't an industry I will be involved in much longer. I am currently completing a MSc degree in Counselling and hope to make a difference to people's lives in that role.

'It's hard to give advice, but I would say, prioritise self-care and don't be afraid to use your voice, even when it seems that it will go unheard.'

RACHEL

'I have been a social worker for ten years and have worked in most areas, as well as with CAFCASS. I am now a manager.

'The major challenges of the work for me are the amount of paperwork and bureaucracy, the heavy caseloads and having to work outside of contractual hours. Often, especially when dealing with young people who live out of county, you can't adopt the collaborative approach that is necessary to give them the time they need. You are often relying on other professionals who are ill equipped and/or give up. I hope to stay in a managerial role so that I can attempt to effect change, as I believe this is the best place to do that.

'My advice to newly qualified social workers would be to read widely, be organised, ask as many questions as possible, ensure that you have a proper induction and a mentor from within your team. Take part in every social work team possible to gain as much experience of young people's journeys so that you adopt an empathetic approach.'

Top tips

Here are my top tips for staying resilient and preparing yourself for a life beyond social work:

1. Accept that the demands of the job will always be high, and resources will always be limited. Try to come to terms

PREPARING YOURSELF

with this so that you don't become dissatisfied and cynical.

2. Remember why you wanted to become a social worker in the first place and keep a sense of purpose and fulfilment in your day-to-day work. Even 'boring paperwork' can make a massive difference to someone's life.

3. Remind yourself how far you have come from your university application to study social work. You have come through that rigorous training and are now living the dream you had then. Be proud of your achievement.

4. Celebrate your achievements, however small, whether making a breakthrough with a client or simply organising your day.

5. Keep pushing yourself and learning, as this will lead to greater fulfilment and confidence, as well as competence.

6. Set yourself goals to aim for so that you don't get stuck in a rut or feel that you are 'going nowhere'.

7. Support and encourage your colleagues, who will then likely do the same for you, making you feel respected and valued.

8. Associate with positive people. If your team is full of negative people, look for a new role.//
9. Be kind to yourself. Don't expect yourself to be perfect, as nobody is, but be content to do your best.
10. Look after yourself, as you cannot look after others otherwise.

Summary

As well as sharpening your social work skills, you must develop yourself to achieve a work/life balance and prepare for a career away from the frontline. This process starts with another greatly underrated practice, self-evaluation, which should become a matter of routine and a subconscious habit.

Constant training and learning, above and beyond what is required of you, should also be part of your programme of self-development. Look out for opportunities for self-improvement that might stand you in good stead as you go forward.

All this will require discipline, which is yet another underrated skill if you are to avoid stress, anxiety and burnout. Learn to recognise the signs of burnout before it happens and take steps to prevent it. For example, drink lots of water, take regular breaks, exercise daily and, above all, get plenty of sleep.

Your aim should be to 'find your why': your purpose in life and what you want to achieve, who you want to be and what legacy you want to leave. This will enable you to create a vision and bring it to fruition, which is the subject of Part Two of this book.

PART TWO
OPPORTUNITIES

The first part of this book essentially discussed what they don't teach you or tell you in the lecture room at university. These are things that you find out for yourself once you qualify, the types of things I am sure thousands of social workers will tell you they wish they had been told about before: strategies for better planning and organisation, for managing stress and avoiding burnout. How to face and overcome the challenges and the pain points. Understanding and implementing legislation, policy and protocols.

SOCIAL WORK AND BEYOND

Talking to social workers, I get the feeling that many of them feel that there is no other option. They cannot see beyond their current position. They think that they are stuck in a bubble and don't know where else they could go. In this second part, I aim to inspire you to look at your skillset and at the opportunities that are open to you both within and beyond social work and to show you how to get there.

It is not my aim to persuade you to leave the social work profession. On the contrary, I will be encouraging you to remain in the sector, but to branch out and set up your own business within it.

As we have seen, there is a growing concern that supported accommodation and residential children's homes are being set up with private equity and other investment funds by people who do not have relevant experience, let alone the necessary attitude towards social care, but are merely out to make money. My aim is to change that narrative by demonstrating that it is possible for those already in the industry to take charge and really make a difference. To move from frontline to CEO in an organic way, without having to 'sell your soul' to investors who are past caring.

FOUR
Taking The Leap

While my aim in this book is not to persuade you to leave social work, the fact is that of the 120,000 or so registered social workers in England, at least 5,000 are now leaving the profession every year. (The figure for 2022 was around 5,400.)[14] While other sources are asking what can be done to stop so many leaving, I am more concerned here with exploring the options available should you, indeed, be considering leaving your current role.

Social work is a world-renowned profession, so as a social worker you have considerable 'value' in the job market. But first, you need to ascertain whether you are ready and willing to move in a new direction, have a vision of where you want to end up, and, if so, how your hard-won skills might be transferable either within the social care sector or outside of it. Then we can explore some of the opportunities that are open to you and what it will take to make that bold leap.

Have I reached my ceiling?

You may be (and most likely are) unhappy about certain aspects of your job as a social worker, but how do you know whether you have reached your ceiling and need to move on?

Obviously, if you are suffering from burnout, that is a sign that a change of occupation is needed. But there are other indications you should be on the lookout for. Is your performance dropping? Are you no longer able to produce the quality of work that you once did? Is your work/life balance swinging in favour of work and beginning to have an impact on you as an individual? If the answers to these questions are yes, it is probably time for you to re-evaluate your future career.

This does not necessarily mean leaving the social care sector altogether. If you are still passionate about the profession, you can divert yourself to other areas within it and these don't have to be mainstream social work. One possibility is to open a business that is related to social work, such as supported accommodation or a residential children's home, both of which are big 'markets' within social care. Another avenue is a social work consultancy, which includes counselling and mentoring.

Of course, you can leave the profession completely and start a career in an entirely new sector. Admittedly, this will require upskilling or reskilling and learning an entirely different subject area, but, as we will see, your many social work skills (outlined in Chapter 2) are highly transferable.

Do I have a vision?

Before you take the leap, it is essential to have a vision of where you want to 'land'; otherwise, you are literally leaping in the dark. So, before you do anything else, write down your vision. Describe it in words and make it as clear and concise as possible. What exactly do you want to achieve? Where do you see yourself in the short- and long-term?

Without a vision, there is no direction. Your vision should show you what you need to do and when, what your goals are for Year 1, Year 2, and so on. This helps you to break down your plan into manageable segments. Your vision should be linked to your interests, knowledge and experience, so my assumption in this book is that as a qualified and possibly experienced social worker, you will want to remain in the social care arena.

Are my skills transferable?

We talked in Chapter 2 about the skills required of a social worker, including communication, planning, organisation and prioritisation, time management and resilience. Typically, therefore, social workers have a large number of transferable skills that are applicable to many types of roles:

- **Interpersonal skills:** You are adept at navigating social situations, both positive and negative. Your ability to understand others' needs, be compassionate, have patience and resolve conflicts will be extremely important in any career you decide to pursue.

- **Communication skills:** Public speaking, negotiating, active listening and effective writing are communication skills that you use regularly and are transferable to many different career fields.

- **Critical thinking skills:** You help others solve problems and rely on your critical thinking skills to analyse situations and make logical decisions. These skills are also easily transferable to alternative jobs.

- **Organisational skills:** Managing documents, schedules and prioritising tasks are organisational skills that many employers outside social work will be looking for.

- **Technical skills:** Your proficiency at basic computer skills such as maintaining a digital database and producing reports and information sheets is also valuable in a variety of alternative careers – especially if you have kept them up to date.

These skillsets can easily be transferred to alternative careers such as school counsellor/safeguarding lead, policy analyst/political assistant, human resources officer or life coach. It is a question of assessing them and 'angling' them towards the demands of your chosen role. Here, though, I want to focus on starting a business within the social work world, where your skills will be most relevant and useful.

Investing in yourself

Importantly, as a social worker you are so much more than a set of skills. You have passion and commitment, you have empathy and understanding, you have determination and a strong work ethic. You are disciplined and resilient. You are knowledgeable and hungry for learning. And now that you have read Chapter 3, you are confident in your own abilities.

In other words, you are your greatest asset, because nobody knows you like you do. But, like any asset, you need constant 'investment' to maintain your 'market value'. Investing in yourself will not only equip you with new knowledge and skills, but also boost your confidence and increase your self-esteem.

Technology and workplaces are changing faster than ever before. Expanding and updating your skillset will ensure that you are ready to adapt to these changes. People with transferable skills are viewed as more flexible, motivated and forward-thinking by both colleagues and superiors. Embracing lifelong learning will also help you achieve a growth mindset and build the resilience needed to navigate life's inevitable challenges and adversities.

Signing up for a new course, workshop or activity will help you grow your network and meet like-minded people. Over time, these relationships can turn into business opportunities or collaborations. It is important to note that, as well as investing in yourself, you should invest in your relationships. Networking is most successful when you approach it with a reciprocal mindset that sees benefits for both parties, rather than just focusing on what is in it for you.

The mental stimulation provided by challenging yourself to learn new skills also promotes brain health and lowers your risk of mental health problems, while focusing on your personal development will help you get to know yourself better. You will become more aware of your unique set of strengths, values and passions and how you can use these to achieve your goals. Investing in yourself should, therefore, be at the top of your priority list.

What are my options?

It is important to remember that social workers can progress both vertically and horizontally. Vertical progression means moving up the career ladder to higher-level positions, while horizontal progression means that you may take on different roles or responsibilities within your current role. So, when you consider your social work career path and how to develop this, it is important to consider your 'why'.

Vertical career progression

As you progress through the ranks, it is very likely you will have less of a frontline role and move more into team or people management. If this appeals to you, then this could be possible in around three to five years after qualification. Your options would likely be to become a senior practitioner or team manager, resulting in a less 'hands-on' role in terms of contact with service users and, instead, an increased responsibility for managing other social workers, as well as involvement in financial and political issues.

Horizontal career progression

Social work offers job roles in many different areas: community services; hospital-based practice; mental health; education; family services; research; administration and management. Each of these areas offers different ways for you to build your skills, knowledge and experience over time so that you can become more specialised in your field – leading ultimately to promotion.

Starting your own business

Your other option – and the one I will be advocating in the rest of this book – is to start your own business, if this interests you. Chapter 5 will discuss the options for starting a business within social care, which is what I have done (twice) and Chapter 6 will look at the nitty-gritty of creating a successful business. I will be looking at three areas in particular: starting a consultancy business, providing supported accommodation, and opening a residential children's home.

Consultancy

Consulting can be a viable option for social workers who want to have more flexibility, autonomy and income potential. Consulting is a form of self-employment that involves providing advice, guidance or training to social workers on specific issues or goals.

You might think that social workers won't be able to afford independent social work consultancy services, but many of them recognise the need for it and are happy to pay to absorb the material and gain insights into coping with the challenges of their job. Just as an entrepreneur might engage a business coach or other busy people invest in personal trainers and life coaches, so social workers are reaching out to consultants to enhance their performance and career prospects. Many people realise that they want more from their jobs, their careers, their lives – and are prepared to pay for it.

The first step to becoming a consultant is to identify the specific area of social work that you are most passionate about and where you have the most experience and knowledge. This will help you define what you can offer your potential clients. Known as your 'value proposition', this is what sets you apart from other consultants – in other words, how you can fill a gap or address a need. For example, you might decide to specialise in working with children, refugees or those suffering substance abuse or trauma. You should also research the market to ascertain the likely demand for your services, the competition you will be facing and the opportunities for expansion and development.

The second step is to decide how to present yourself and your services to your target audience (known as building your brand). Your brand should reflect your chosen area of specialism (your niche), your values and your personality. You will need to create a professional image that conveys a sense of expertise, credibility and trustworthiness. Your brand should be consistent across your website, logo, business cards and any social media presence.

The third step to becoming a consultant is to set your rates, ie, how much you will charge for your services. You will need to consider how much you want to earn, how much you will need to invest in your business, and how much your clients are willing or able to pay. You should also decide on your billing method – whether you will charge by the hour or per project or ask for a retainer.

As a consultant, you must plan, organise and execute your projects effectively and efficiently, and meet your deadlines and expectations. You should also monitor and evaluate your outcomes and report them to your clients regularly. You should be flexible and adaptable to changing needs and situations and be ready to solve problems and overcome challenges.

You will, of course, need to keep learning and updating your skills, and stay on top of the latest trends, research and best practices in your niche. You should seek feedback from clients and use this to enhance your services. You should also pursue professional development opportunities such as courses, certifications, workshops and conferences that can help you develop your expertise and expand your network.

Bear in mind that while consulting can be rewarding, it can also be demanding and stressful. You will need to take care of yourself and avoid burnout by setting boundaries, prioritising tasks, delegating work and outsourcing support. You should also maintain a healthy lifestyle by eating well, sleeping enough, exercising regularly, relaxing often and spending quality time with your family, friends, and community.

But you already do all those things, don't you?

Supported accommodation

As children grow up and approach adulthood, they gradually gain more independence from their parents – a transition that the care system seeks to replicate. Until the age of sixteen, most looked-after children in the care system are best placed in foster care or in a children's home, but at sixteen they can move to supported accommodation if they are ready for it.

Supported accommodation, as the name indicates, provides accommodation with support for sixteen- and seventeen-year-old looked-after children and care leavers to enable them to live semi-independently. The aim of supported accommodation is to support young people to develop independence in preparation for adult living while keeping them safe in a homely and nurturing environment.

Over the last few years, large numbers of social workers have started businesses offering supported accommodation. Historically, it was viewed as the simplest first step for those wanting to transition from social work, as setting up supported accommodation was unregulated and, therefore, a seamless process. This resulted in the market becoming saturated, with individuals such as landlords without direct experience in social work profiting from sub-standard accommodation with little or no support.

However, on 28th April 2023, Ofsted began registering supported accommodation providers and registration became mandatory on 28th October 2023. This means that any provider accommodating a looked-after child or care leaver aged sixteen or seventeen must either be registered with Ofsted or have had an application accepted by Ofsted as complete before 28th October 2023. The new regulations include mandatory quality standards in supported accommodation and an inspection regime.

Nevertheless, due to the traditional popularity of setting up a supported accommodation business, there is still a considerable amount of competition and a lot to take on board in terms of administrative procedures and strategies.

The first thing to do, once you have decided to take the leap, is to register your new company with Companies House. Then you must work out your budget and make a twelve-month financial forecast. The third – and hardest – thing to do is to find a suitable property. (We will look at this in more detail below.) Bear in mind that you cannot register with Ofsted without a property, and you cannot tender for contracts until you are registered. As with any property, location is key, but you will want it to be somewhere you can commute to quickly and easily. A location risk assessment will need to be completed for each premises.

Regarding budgeting, it is important to remember that you will normally have to pay up to six months' rent upfront, before you have an income, as this is how long the registration and referral process can take. You will also need to furnish the property and cover your startup costs, so you will need a lot of resilience and perseverance, as well as financial resources.

As a social worker you are unlikely to have this amount of money in your piggy bank to invest in a business, so you will need either to obtain a bank loan or to find investors – the preferred option. We will look at strategies for finding investors in Chapter 5.

Residential children's homes

The other option I would like to discuss here is opening a residential children's home, offering nurturing and therapeutic care for children and young people between the ages of about eight and seventeen. Because of the level of care required, this is a more complex and costly option which requires both more resources and more energy, but one that, in my opinion, potentially offers greater rewards.

Having owned supported accommodation, I have found it preferable to work with younger children because you have more scope to develop and empower them and to map their future than you do with young people of sixteen or seventeen. Your aim is to create a safe space, a nurturing environment in which these young people can thrive, and to prepare them to take the bold leap from a traumatic childhood to independent adulthood. To do this, you need to engage them and equip them with sensible, practical, reliable knowledge, insights, routines and patterns of behaviour.

Looking back, I wish that I had started with a residential children's home rather than with supported accommodation, but this would have been more difficult, especially as I was working full-time while trying to start a business.

As with supported accommodation, you will need to register your business with both Companies House and Ofsted and find a suitable property. In the case of a residential children's home, however, your biggest challenges will be finding the working capital and recruiting the right staff. Partly for this reason, but also because the registration process for a residential children's home is much longer (it can take up to six months), you are looking at a startup budget of around £150,000, depending on whether you will be leasing a property or purchasing and developing.

What will it take?

Whichever direction you decide to take, you should be under no illusions as to how difficult it will be. There will be no overnight success in any field. It will be a long and sometimes arduous journey, and you will have to give it time. So, the first thing to do is to acknowledge and accept this, and to recognise that there are reasons for this.

If you are thinking of setting up your own business, you will almost certainly not be able to 'simply' walk out of your job, unless you have considerable independent financial means. However dissatisfied you are with your present job, you must not let your emotions get the better of you and give in to a 'knee-jerk' reaction by handing in your notice as soon as you have made your decision to move on.

There must necessarily be a transition period (in my case, it was three years) during which you will have to continue working full-time as a social worker while you establish your business and develop it to the stage at which it is making sufficient profit to support you (and your family if that applies). This will be tough. I know, because I have done it. As you know only too well, social work is rarely a nine-to-five job. You will often have to work longer hours while still trying to find the time to start something new and get it off the ground. This will require grit and determination, patience and self-belief. Believe me.

You will also need to plan carefully, without underestimating the time you will need to put everything in place that is necessary for your new business to succeed. However long it takes, you must always keep your end goal in mind: freeing yourself from the stresses and strains of social work and becoming your own boss. It is a bold leap, but one you will not regret. After twelve years as a social worker thinking, 'What else can I do? This is all I know,' I took that leap and I have never looked back.

Summary

As a result of your self-evaluation and self-development strategy you will know whether you have 'reached your ceiling' and have a vision of where you want to go. You have a variety of valuable skills and a precious asset: yourself. Several options are therefore open to you.

If you choose to stay within the social care sector as I recommend, then you can set up as a consultant or coach, you can provide supported accommodation or you can open a residential children's home.

Independent consultants are increasingly in demand by social workers and recognised by local authorities as providing a valuable service to social workers, who are prepared to pay to improve their effectiveness and wellbeing.

Supported accommodation is a popular 'first step' for those wanting to move up from frontline social work – and for this reason, an increasingly competitive environment, so careful research and budgeting is a must before you take the leap.

Setting up a residential children's home requires even more meticulous planning, since it is strictly regulated by Ofsted, but can be even more rewarding in terms of empowering children and young people to take their place in society.

Whichever route you decide to take, you can be sure that there will be no overnight success; establishing a business takes time and requires patience, determination and self-belief.

FIVE
Making It Happen

One skill you may not have as a social worker is setting up and running a business. There are, of course, numerous books on the subject. In this chapter, I will focus on the essentials as they relate to starting a business in the social care sector. These are market research, branding and online visibility, recruitment, finances, premises and the legalities.

I have said before (and make no apology for repeating it here) that there will be no overnight success. Starting a business in any field requires hard work, commitment and perseverance. A social care business is no exception.

Knowing the market

If you are starting a consultancy or opening supported accommodation or a residential children's home as I have suggested, you will, of course, already have a good knowledge of the social work market and how it works, what the requirements are, where the needs and opportunities lie and what the current and likely future trends are. Nevertheless, before committing yourself to any business, you should carry out detailed market research to ascertain whether there is a need for it, and if it is likely to be viable.

As well as 'book' (and internet) research, this will involve talking to people in the relevant area. I also strongly recommend that you consult a business coach who has knowledge and experience in that area and understands the business structures, systems and processes that will work best for you.

Achieving visibility

Visibility is the frequency which your business (or 'brand') is seen on different marketing channels, as opposed to brand awareness, which is the extent to which people are familiar with your business. Businesses with greater visibility also tend to have better brand awareness, but this isn't always the case. To build awareness, you need high visibility, ie, repeated interactions with your target audience.

To achieve this, you might also consider engaging a marketing and brand consultant. Although marketing is not really a requirement in the social care sector, since your client base is well-defined and limited (social workers if you are a consultant and local authorities if you are setting up supported accommodation or a residential children's home), you will, nevertheless, need to create a positive image, have high online visibility and generate a good reputation, all of which requires skills that you might not have.

After all, as a social worker you are used to putting others first rather than 'blowing your own trumpet', as you will need to do to create a successful business out of nothing. A good and reputable brand consultant will not only ensure that you have an excellent website that is high on search lists, but also create a distinctive and recognisable 'brand' for you and establish you as an authority in your area.

Regarding reputation, however, keep in mind that in the supported accommodation and children's home sector, this will hinge on your Ofsted grading. Achieving an 'outstanding' grade will be worth more than any amount of advertising or PR, because everyone will automatically know that your services are of high quality. Conversely, if your Ofsted grading is 'requires improvement', no amount of billboard advertising, YouTube videos, leaflet drops, emails or LinkedIn posts will overturn the inspection result.

With high visibility and a solid reputation, you should find that you are literally turning business away. This is especially true in the social care sector, where you are dealing with vulnerable children and young people and your clients, first and foremost, want to be sure that you are who you say you are and that you are providing the best possible service.

Visibility and reputation will also help you with recruitment, since people will come to you asking you to employ them (as has happened to me more than once).

One caveat regarding visibility in the case of a children's home is, of course, that the location of the property should remain 'invisible' for safeguarding reasons. In that case, it is your 'head office' address that should be visible (and respectable).

Assembling a team

You will soon realise that you cannot do everything by yourself; as John Donne famously wrote, 'No man is an island...'[15] One of the most common mistakes entrepreneurs make is to think that they can 'go it alone'. As has been proven time and again, it is simply not possible. The one-man band is generally a recipe for disaster. They might survive for a year or two – though often at great cost to their health and wellbeing but, ultimately, they are doomed to failure.

You must accept the fact that you will need help, but not just any help. A key to the success of any business startup is building a power team, which goes way beyond the necessity of hiring. This step involves vision and intent to create an internal support structure made up of people who really 'get' your company and its principles and aims. To make it a success, they must be excited about what you have created and committed to investing in it. You are the entrepreneur, and your team members are the 'intrapreneurs'. Assembling such a team will result in the right environment, the right culture, which is a vital ingredient of any successful business.

Once again, finding the right people is a matter of talking to the right people, networking and building relationships. I attended a Business Network International (BNI) event in Birmingham and I was introduced to an accountant, a branding consultant and an IT consultant. That's how I got started.

Working out the finances

One of your biggest challenges will inevitably be money or, rather, the lack of it. But, as they say, 'Where there's a will there's a way,' and you should never let finances be an obstacle to achieving your dream.

First, you must be realistic. We have talked about the sort of money you will need to start supported accommodation or a residential children's home. Don't, however, assume that these will be your actual costs. Work it out for yourself and prepare a detailed forecast with a healthy contingency built in. This is a very important part of mapping your business strategy and achieving your goals.

Before you go looking for funding, you must be confident not only in your numbers but also in your product, your brand and your business model. Do your research, carry out your due diligence. Nobody will part with money to help you unless you can convince them that you will be able to at least repay them and, preferably, return them a dividend.

To raise this initial capital, you have several options. The conventional method is to borrow it – to take out a loan that you agree to repay over a set period. Mainstream banks may also offer you an overdraft facility with an agreed amount of loan finance that is available to manage your cash flow when you need it. I took out a loan with Nationwide Finance to finance my first startup and this was simple and straightforward, so I would advise you not to be afraid of taking out a business loan.

Another option is to ask people you know or who support you personally for financial support. For example, a group of friends and/or family members might each lend you £1,000 to get your organisation up and running.

Another possibility is finding investors who are willing to make an investment in exchange for shares in your organisation. For example, an investor might pay £10,000 to own 10% of your organisation. Equity investors receive a share of any profits paid out by your organisation and get to have a say in how it is run, proportionate to the amount they have invested.

To find investors, you will need to be creative, resourceful and persistent. It takes time and there are no short-cuts. You will also realise that there are different types of investors. So, having an early idea of what you want from them will benefit you in the long run. Though it might be tempting to take the first offer you receive, don't! Meet several investors. The right ones will give you more than money; they will also bring experience, passion, an understanding of your sector, guidance and even friendship.

Meanwhile, potential investors will want you to tell them what makes your business stand out. They will be seeking a story, a vision they can buy into, so you will need to produce a pitch deck (and rehearse it thoroughly with people you know). Remember that you are not simply interviewing potential investors; they are interviewing you.

On average, it takes six months to find an investor and secure a deal. When I started my first business, in August 2020, I had to continue doing social work for nearly three years until, eventually, in March 2023, I was able to exit the profession and focus on my business full time.

This means that you cannot simply 'throw in the towel' in your current job and hope to have your business up and running before your savings dry up. You must have a plan that maps out a phased transition from social worker to entrepreneur. It is about sacrificing the here and now for the rewards you are going to reap down the line. As the cliché goes, 'No gain without pain.'

Making a profit

Like any business, yours needs to make a profit. Profit is the fuel that keeps it going and helps it to grow. Without profit, your business will eventually fail. It doesn't matter how small or big your business is; every company needs to make a profit to survive and thrive. But profit is not just about numbers on a balance sheet; it is about having the resources available when they are needed. This could be when you need to hire new staff or invest in a marketing campaign.

Profit is a somewhat contentious issue in the social care sector, as there are those who argue that no one should profit from local authorities, but that all the money should go towards the provision of care. The recent paper 'Profit Making and Risk in Independent Children's Social Care Placement Providers',[16] compiled in response to Competition and Markets Authority (CMA) reporting, revealed that big social care companies running homes for children are making average profit margins of 19%, which has caused an uproar in certain circles.[17]

Profitability is, however, a sign that the company is providing a good service and, hopefully, reinvesting some of those profits in the care of young people in need by, for example, purchasing new premises and land on which to construct new properties, engaging additional staff, training those staff to higher standards and increasing their salaries accordingly.

'Profit with purpose' is a foundation for growth and security. Local Authorities have even recognised that specialisms of care have been developed in the independent sector that could not easily have been developed within the public sphere.

The question of profitability relates back to the issue of self-care, which we discussed in Chapter 2. Just as you cannot look after others if you don't first look after yourself, so you will not be able to provide effective care services unless you are running an effective, ie, profitable, business.

Finding premises

Another major challenge you must face is finding premises for your supported accommodation or residential children's home. If you are renting a property, which is probable as you are unlikely to be able to afford to buy premises, at least initially, you will have to find a landlord who will buy into your vision and be happy for their property to be used for children or young people in care, which not all are. This means that you may need to devote a lot of time and effort to contacting, pitching to and building relationships with landlords, developers and letting agents.

An alternative is to work with private property investors, who often have a wide range of skills and experience to help you find the property you need and to get it set up quickly. They often have local connections to help them source property that may not be on the open market. Building relationships with property investors can also help you grow your business, since many of them are looking to build a supported living property portfolio.

If you decide to approach investors, make it clear what type of property you need and help them to understand your requirements. This can save you considerable time and stress. Bear in mind, however, that property investors are often very creative and can adapt and change a property that you may have discounted as being unsuitable.

Many property investors can also support you when it comes to property compliance. There are many things to consider such as EPC, gas and electrical safety checks, HMO licensing and regulation. Property compliance is complicated and fast-changing, so having a trusted partner who is up to date on these issues can be a big time-saver.

When I started my company in 2020, I opened four supported accommodation locations within the first twelve months because suitable properties became available, which was simply crazy. With hindsight, I would have paced myself, which is why I advise you to do the same.

In the case of a children's home, there is the added complication of needing to obtain planning permission from the local authority to use the premises as such. Getting planning permission is no simple matter. All planning applications are considered in relation to the Council's adopted Development Plan (Local Plan), which sets out policies for different types of development. Sometimes there is a separate policy for care homes and sometimes it is covered by a general policy. Other regulations and guidelines can also be relevant, such as national policy and ministerial statements. Note that in London there is also the London Plan, which takes precedence over the Local Plans of the individual boroughs.

I therefore strongly suggest seeking professional planning advice from a chartered town planner before proceeding with an application. They can help you appraise a property to see what planning issues you might face and whether your application might be successful. They can also advise you on what information should be provided with an application.

Negotiating the legalities

Before you can open supported accommodation or a residential children's home, you must satisfy the authorities, specifically Ofsted, that you will be providing adequate accommodation and meeting all the relevant regulations and standards.

As of 28th October 2023, all care providers in England offering housing and support (supported accommodation) to sixteen- and seventeen-year-old looked-after children and care leavers must register with Ofsted. The requirement addresses long-standing concerns over the sector's lack of regulation and aims to ensure the safety and wellbeing of these vulnerable individuals. Running such a service without registration is now an offence. The Supported Accommodation (England) Regulations 2023[18] introduced four Quality Standards, which all registered providers must comply with: the leadership and management standard, the protection standard, the accommodation standard, and the support standard. Together, these ensure that accommodation provides safe living conditions, has effective governance, effectively safeguards residents and provides personalised support plans.

Ofsted is also responsible for ensuring that your business complies with the Children's Homes Regulations,[19] brought into force in April 2015, with the aim of ensuring that such homes provide adequate care, protection and positive development.

Ofsted inspections can be both painful and nerve-wracking, but you can minimise the anxiety and the risk of negative consequences by preparing thoroughly for them. This means checking your objectives and your KPIs to ensure that they are on point, reviewing your leadership and management structure and making sure that every member of your team is doing what they need to be doing. Ensure, of course, that you are keeping children safe and achieving the desired educational or activity-based outcomes and, above all, evidencing that.

The importance of providing evidence of everything you are doing, including the progress each child has made, the challenges you have faced and how you have overcome them and the training and upskilling you have given your staff cannot be overstated.

Summary

For all your skills as a social worker, you may not know how to set up and run a business. You must first research your market, if necessary, with the help of a business consultant. Then you must work on your image and create an identity or 'brand' for your business, which will make you 'visible' and build you a good reputation.

You cannot run a business by yourself, so you will need to assemble a 'power team' of experts and specialists that you can rely on. This means getting out there and networking and talking to the people you intend to engage.

Raising capital will be your next big challenge and you have various options, including friends and family, banks and investors. This takes time, which means that you might need to continue practising as a social worker for up to three years while you establish your business.

Then, if you are opening supported accommodation or a children's home, you must find premises and negotiate the legalities, including meeting Ofsted regulations and standards.

It's a lot of work, but it will be worth it as we shall see in the final chapter.

SIX
Living Your Purpose

In this final chapter, I would like to look at the rewards, the payoff for all the hard work and sacrifice you will have put into achieving your goal; to remind you of your purpose in doing so and show you that you can live that purpose.

At the start of your journey to this point, you evaluated yourself and found your why and what you were really interested in, what you were good at, what your skills were, your strengths and your weaknesses. You reflected on the reasons you came into social work in the first place – to be an agent of change, to enhance the lives of others, to give a voice to the voiceless in society. You examined your social work practice, your experiences and the challenges you had faced and overcome. You implemented strategies to improve your practice within the profession and prepare yourself for the next stage in your career. You considered the options open to you, both within and outside social work. You opened your horizons and thought on a larger scale about what you wanted going forwards. Then you created a vision and put together a plan and, finally, you executed that plan and delivered on your vision.

Now you can, and deserve to, enjoy the satisfaction of having achieved your ambition to start your own business or take your career to another level, the fulfilment of being your own boss and controlling your own destiny.

Enjoy the challenge(s)

When I decided to stop practising as a social worker in March 2023 to devote myself full-time to my own business, I felt a deep sense of satisfaction and gratification. I felt content; I felt whole. Of course, I then faced a new set of challenges, but I realised that what I had achieved empowered me to deal with those challenges. Having achieved my purpose, I was able to navigate the tides and ride the waves that came my way.

One of the biggest challenges you will face in starting your own business is adaptation and altering your mindset from that of a practitioner on the frontline within social work, dealing with crisis intervention and safeguarding issues, with data and with KPIs, with the here and now, to that of a CEO, having to think about business management, about staffing, about raising capital, marketing and branding, about strategic planning and forecasting and overseeing the operation of a business. These are very different worlds, and your success will depend very much on your ability to adapt and invest in personal development. You may have achieved your goal, but there is no question of putting your feet up. You must keep on learning, evolving and investing in yourself.

As we have seen (in Chapter 2), however, the skills you have developed as a social worker – above all, your ability to problem-solve and achieve outcomes – will equip you to deal with these new challenges. You will also be well used to learning on the job, to being proactive and taking responsibility for important decisions.

Yes, you have done a degree in social work, but running a business is completely different. Hence, it is important that you surround yourself with a power team of people who have the knowledge and expertise you lack.

Where you might previously have felt stuck in a rut, merely trying to keep your head above water, the very fact that you have new challenges to face and new obstacles to overcome will give you renewed energy and job-satisfaction.

Your new position will also open new opportunities. I began by opening a supported accommodation business and soon realised that what I really wanted to do was start a residential children's home, which I probably could not have done, or even envisaged, had I not taken the intermediate step of running supported accommodation. Beyond that, I have discovered that I can now help others to do what I have done by writing this book and by talking on the subject at workshops and seminars.

Perhaps most importantly, I have experienced benefits to my health and wellbeing. I now have less stress and anxiety, and more time for myself and my family. To put it simply, I enjoy life a lot more.

Let go of the reins

You might be thinking, 'I've just taken on the responsibility of running my own business; how on earth can I "let go of the reins"?' But one of the essential differences between being a frontline social worker and being a CEO is that you no longer do everything yourself. In fact, you mustn't. One of the biggest mistakes you can make in starting your own business is thinking that you should do everything and that, because you are in charge, you must have control of all aspects of the business. This will lead to more stress, anxiety and burnout. It is a recipe for disaster – as so many entrepreneurs have found to their cost.

You have assembled a power team; they know what they are doing, so let them. Delegate tasks that they will perform better than you, leaving yourself free to oversee, to plan and direct. That is your role now. You no longer need to run around like the proverbial headless chicken, as you did before.

Nor does the buck always need to stop with you, as it did. In delegating, you will make others accountable, so that responsibility is shared and the pressure on your shoulders is lightened. You can trust them and truly work as a team, which provides its own satisfaction.

Take your time

We have already learned that it takes time to make the transition from social worker to CEO. To progress from startup to established business usually takes around three years. Your business must find its feet and be generating consistent revenue before you can hand in your notice and start your new life as CEO. It doesn't happen overnight, but requires patience and perseverance.

Even having taken the leap, you shouldn't expect to enjoy plain sailing from the word go, but should allow yourself another eighteen or twenty-four months to reach the point where your business is making sufficient profit to establish itself in the market.

This was my experience and during that period I had a lot of doubts. Had I made the right decision? Was I doing things right? Would it work? Should I continue? Was this really for me? This is where you will need to call on your resilience and, above all, not be too hard on yourself if you feel that you aren't achieving your targets within the anticipated time. If you truly believe in your vision and keep going, you will get there sooner or later.

Trust the process

If, like me, you are faced with doubts, it is important to keep faith in your vision and trust the process of achieving it. Take the time to periodically check in with that vision. Remind yourself of your purpose, of what you want to achieve and why, to restore your belief in yourself and the people around you and strengthen your resolve not to give up.

It is not an easy road from a social worker to CEO. If it was, everyone would be taking it, so trusting in the process is critical to your success.

Create a legacy

Inherent in the process of starting a business is creating something that will outlast you, that will continue to have an impact in the world after you are gone. This is another important consideration that should sustain you in moments of doubt or uncertainty.

Always remember that your business isn't just for you, nor even for your family or descendants. It is for the young people and children who are in your care. It is about the impact it will have on their lives as they develop and grow into adults. This will be your true legacy and a worthwhile and invaluable one.

As we have seen, the social care sector in the UK is being 'invaded' by big businesses that, in fact, care little for those in their care but are more concerned with making money. As a social worker, you will be able to buck that trend and create a business founded on the principles of social work, which will hopefully show the right way forward to those that follow you.

Summary

The rewards for all your hard work in setting up a business will be many and, perhaps, unexpected. You will, of course, face new challenges, but they will be enjoyable challenges, since you will be able to share them with your team and know that you will benefit from overcoming them.

Perhaps the greatest challenge, however, will be adapting your attitude and approach from that of a frontline practitioner to that of a forward-thinking 'director of operations'. Once again, however, you will have a team of experts around you to help you make this transition.

Once you have made it, you will be able to 'let go the reins' and enjoy being your own boss. It will take time but, if you trust the process, you will achieve your goal and realise your vision – which will not only give you great satisfaction, but also open other opportunities you might not have anticipated such as helping others to achieve what you have achieved.

Finally, of course, you will have something to leave as a legacy and a lasting contribution to the profession you joined with such golden ideals and passion.

Conclusion

Social workers support people in a variety of ways. They play a crucial role in facilitating change and development, and advocate for a fairer society by tackling inequality. They provide a voice for those that need it and promote the human rights and wellbeing of those they support. This is why we need social work to be the best profession it can be.

A career in social work, however, presents great challenges, which I hope you will be better equipped to meet and overcome because of implementing the strategies outlined in this book – honing your skills and developing yourself so as to be more competent and perform to the best of your ability.

You should also be more aware of the importance of looking after yourself, of the indicators of burnout and of the signs that you have reached your ceiling and are ready to move on by starting your own business, whether within or outside the social work sector.

You now know what your options are, have a vision of where you want to go and realise what it takes to get there. It is not easy and cannot be achieved overnight, but if I can do it, I am confident that you can too. I wish you every success and happiness.

Notes

1. E Munro, N Cartwright, J Hardie and E Montuschi, 'Improving Child Safety: Deliberation, judgement and empirical research' (Centre for Humanities Engaging Science and Society, 2016), www.durham.ac.uk/media/durham-university/research-/research-centres/humanities-engaging-sci-and-soc-centre-for/ONLINE_Improvingchildsafety-15_2_17-FINAL.pdf, accessed 20 March 2024
2. Department of Education, Working Together to Safeguard Children (Gov.UK, 2023), https://assets.publishing.service.gov.uk/media/65cb4349a7ded0000c79e4e1/Working_together_to_safeguard_children_2023_-_statutory_guidance.pdf, accessed 20 March 2024
3. 'Professional Standards' (Social Work England, no date), www.socialworkengland.org.uk/media/1640/1227_socialworkengland_standards_prof_standards_final-aw.pdf, accessed 20 March 2024
4. 'Code of Ethics' (BASW, Jan 2012), https://new.basw.co.uk/policy-practice/standards/code-ethics#Background, accessed 20 March 2024
5. 'The Pomodoro® Technique', The Pomodoro® Technique (no date), www.pomodorotechnique.com/what-is-the-pomodoro-technique.php, accessed 20 March 2024
6. 'The Eisenhower Matrix: Urgent vs important tasks template', Reclaimai (20 October 2022), https://reclaim.ai/blog/eisenhower-matrix, accessed 20 March 2024
7. R Hall, 'Social workers in England quitting in record numbers' (*The Guardian*, 9 February 2023), www.theguardian.com/society/2023/feb/23/social-workers-in-england-quitting-in-record-numbers, accessed 20 March 2024

8. 'Child Safeguarding Practice Review Panel: annual report 2021' (Gov.UK, 15 December 2022), www.gov.uk/government/publications/child-safeguarding-practice-review-panel-annual-report-2021, accessed 20 March 2024
9. 'Burnout' (Mental Health UK, no date), https://mentalhealth-uk.org/burnout, accessed 20 March 2024
10. 'The Burnout Report' (Mental Health UK, January 2024), https://mhukcdn.s3.eu-west-2.amazonaws.com/wp-content/uploads/2024/01/19145241/Mental-Health-UK_The-Burnout-Report-2024.pdf, accessed 20 March 2024
11. 'Over half a million sickness days lost due to mental health issues and work stress in social care' (Social Work News, 20 September 2023), www.mysocialworknews.com/article/over-half-a-million-sickness-days-lost-due-to-mental-health-issues-and-work-stress-in-social-care, accessed 20 March 2024
12. M Söderström, et al, 'Insufficient sleep predicts clinical burnout', J Occup Health Psychol (April 2012), https://doi.org/10.1037/a0027518, accessed 20 March 2024
13. C Hirotsu, et al, 'Interactions between sleep, stress, and metabolism: From physiological to pathological conditions', Sleep Science (November 2015), doi: 10.1016/j.slsci.2015.09.002, accessed 20 March 2024
14. R Hall, 'Social workers in England quitting in record numbers', *The Guardian* (23 February 2023), www.theguardian.com/society/2023/feb/23/social-workers-in-england-quitting-in-record-numbers, accessed 21 March 2024
15. J Donne, Devotions upon Emergent Occasions, Meditation 17 (1624)
16. 'Profit making and risk in independent children's social care placement providers', Local Government Association (no date), www.local.gov.uk/profit-making-and-risk-independent-childrens-social-care-placement-providers, accessed 21 March 2024
17. S Das, 'Private UK care homes' profit margins soared in pandemic, research finds', *The Guardian* (24 July 2022), www.theguardian.com/society/2022/jul/24/uk-private-care-providers-profit-rise-covid-report, accessed 21 March 2024

18. 'The Supported Accommodation (England) Regulations 2023', Legislation.Gov.UK (no date), www.legislation.gov.uk/uksi/2023/416/made, accessed 21 March 2024
19. 'The Children's Homes (England) Regulations 2015', Legislation.Gov.UK (no date), www.legislation.gov.uk/uksi/2015/541/contents/made, accessed 21 March 2024

Acknowledgements

A big thank you to Hon Dr Nsaba Buturo, my father, who taught me to think big. In remembrance of my mother, Mary Buturo, who was an inspiration to me. To Noa Buturo, my daughter, who fills my heart with joy each day. Thank you to Hayley Buturo, my wife, for the countless times you have stood by my side. To my brothers and sister, Daniel Buturo, Apolo Buturo and Jackie Buturo, for the support they provided.

Thank you to my friends, David Hall, Akin Ogunbanjo, Marcel Simpson, Michael Walsh and Michael Thomas, who taught me the true meaning of friendship. To Monica and Fabian

Anderson for their encouragement and unwavering love when I needed it most.

Thank you to Caroline Lee, my personal tutor at Birmingham City University, for the support that enabled me to complete my BSc Hons Social Work degree programme. Thank you to Sharon Pommils for her endless support as Team Manager in what was my first ever qualified social work position at Sandwell Council. A big thank you to all social workers that I had the privilege to work alongside for over ten years. You helped me learn how to survive and thrive in social work.

Thank you to my writing coach, Joe Laredo at Rethink Press, who helped create this exceptional book. To Dr Beverley Barnett-Jones, who provided the Foreword and insightful feedback to help polish my efforts.

The Author

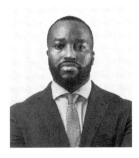

Peter Nduwayesu Buturo is originally from Kampala, Uganda. He lives in Birmingham, England. After obtaining a Bachelor of Science degree in Social Work from Birmingham City University, he embarked upon a career as a social worker and foster carer. In 2020, Peter started his own business and founded Bold Leap, where he provides care and support to children in care within a residential home setting and supported accommodation. *Social Work and Beyond* is his first book. To connect, visit:

in www.linkedin.com/in/peterbuturo
🌐 www.bold-leap.com

(S) 85 - 9/6.

~~Forward~~ contains various refs to business. ✓

Intro.
✗ for social workers.
  ✓ BUT - p8 - "I want more social workers to open their own businesses within social care"

Ch 1. Fascinating and ref to how wanted to do something entrepreneurial as well as social care/work.

Ch 2. Honing your skills. Specific to social
✗ care. Great advice Transferable skills but NO mention of biz.

Ch 3. Good advice for s/workers. No ref
p61 ✗ to biz or a wider career until p74
— p74-81 - Still no ref to biz.

Part 2 - p83.
✓ wonderful ambition → ~~social worker~~
                      → social worker → £60.
                                (in care sector)
Ch 4 p 85
✓ see espec. p 93.
✓ Great advice.

Ch 5 solid
✓ Good business advice.
✗ ~~Doesn't explain all avenues~~ (p116)

Ch 6 ✗ ~~Only~~ ~~just found~~ full
     ✗ Only went full-time into biz March 13
                                    (p124)